FOREST TRAILS TO WELLNESS

FOREST TRAILS TO WELLNESS

WILLIAM VINCENT

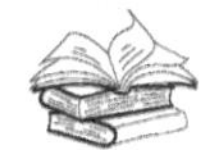

CONTENTS

CHAPTER 1

Introduction to the Healing Power of Nature

Scientific studies confirm that humans cannot thrive when removed from nature. We depend on Earth's diverse species to maintain good health. Natural landscapes are essential for exercise and reducing negative stress. Our built-in preference for looking at nature helps shift attention away from age, chronic illness, and emotional distress. As urban areas expand, it's crucial for people to have urban and rural settings where they can safely enjoy nature's healing power.

Unfortunately, getting outdoors often requires money and leisure time. Many people feel the stress of poverty or unsafe places. Older individuals worry about steep slopes and uneven trails. Those with chronic illnesses might struggle with heat and sun exposure. Injuries and chronic illnesses can make nature inaccessible. People balancing chronic illness repairs and job schedules can find it challenging to arrange transportation to a beautiful location with even pavement. Too often, nature is overlooked because of age, injury, or illness. However, getting outdoors can be uplifting and beneficial to health.

The Physical Benefits of Hiking

Hiking is a healthier option than sitting around. As a society, Americans have started gaining weight in recent years due to lack of movement and a diet filled with fast food. Hiking addresses this problem, providing a healthy activity to help maintain a healthy weight. Unlike working or driving, which can be physically tense, hiking is relaxing. You can meet wonderful people who share your love of nature, find scenic trails, relieve stress, and become healthier both physically and spiritually. Unlike a walk in the park, hiking is a complete mind and body cleansing experience, perfect for relaxation.

You can choose a light stroll on a nicely groomed trail or a more challenging, steep, long trail—it's up to you. Walking on natural ground feels better than pavement, reducing overall physical strain. Advice from letters, newspapers, and other reading materials on maintaining peak physical fitness is correct. Stagnation can lead to major health problems. Now that you understand the importance of preparation and enjoyment of the trail, continue regular excursions throughout the year. These outdoor adventures will keep your emotional spirits healthy. Renewing your connection with nature will immediately improve your mental state. By leaving the house for the trail and enjoying the good things in life, psychological stressors will quickly dissipate. Your body will become accustomed to the trail and start feeling better. Emotional cleansing is bound to follow simple physical exertion on the trail, charging your mind and energizing your body.

Cardiovascular Health

Hiking provides a regular, vigorous workout. When skin temperature rises, the nervous system stimulates sweat glands to produce perspiration, which evaporates to cool the body. Walking for exercise and pleasure can be one of the simplest steps to a healthier heart, especially for overweight individuals. Walking is suitable for practically everyone, particularly the middle-aged and elderly.

Walking has other advantages too. It requires no special tools except comfortable shoes, and it can be done almost anytime and anywhere, in practically any weather. It combines the need for healthful exercise with getting somewhere. Walking to work can save time and money. It takes less time than you might imagine and requires no willpower. It not only changes blood pressure and waistlines but also improves mental attitudes by offering the pleasure of exercise and time for thinking while walking.

Weight Management and Metabolism

The standard American diet (SAD) is rich in processed foods and fast food, contributing to the high prevalence of obesity through high-calorie products containing fat and sugar (soda, sugary fruit drinks, chips, and most meal replacement bars). Obesity is associated with glucose intolerance and insulin resistance. The type of fat consumed can affect obesity, with monounsaturated fats increasing HDL "good" cholesterol and reducing VLDL cholesterol. Obese individuals should reduce fat intake and drink water instead of calorie-containing beverages like soda, sports drinks, fruit drinks, and alcoholic beverages. High glycemic carbohydrates and high-fat, low-fiber diets may reduce insulin sensitivity and increase the incidence of type II diabetes.

Nutrient intake and growth hormone (GH) regulate metabolism. Appropriate nutrient intake is necessary for physical functioning. Insulin-like growth factor-1 (IGF-1) is activated through nutritionally dependent pathways, with reduced expression during starvation and increased expression with GH treatment. Protein malnutrition leads to growth retardation. GH also affects lipoprotein particles and triglyceride-lowering effects in obese adults. Low levels of GH in adult-onset GH-deficiency syndrome relate to qualitative changes in lipoprotein particle metabolism, altering LDL size distribution relative to the control group. These adverse lipoprotein alterations are associated with insulin resistance and increased cardiovascular disease. Iron-deficiency anemia influences an individual's work capacity. GH/IGF-1 interaction inversely relates to muscle catabolism, with decreased availability of IGF-1 in chronic kidney disease patients due to low GH concentrations.

CHAPTER 2

The Mental Health Benefits of Hiking

"Walking through the forest without any goal is an American restorative where a man can lose himself in comfort." – Hal Borland

Regardless of the type of outdoor activity, you usually feel less stress, fewer symptoms of anxiety or depression, and an overall better mood when participating. This aligns with the Attention Restoration Theory and the Stress Reduction Theory, which suggest that time spent in natural environments decreases negative feelings and thoughts, while increasing positive ones. Fresh air and exposure to sunlight, even without a strenuous hike, are nurturing.

Japanese researchers have identified three key factors contributing to nature's restorative effects: the types of odors found in wood, the monotonous sounds created in forests, and the physical activity involved. Studies in Japan have shown that individuals walking through forests exhibit fewer symptoms of negative mood and improved immunity compared to those walking through cities, even at the same average walking speed. Forest walkers experienced a decrease in blood pressure and an increase in the activity of the parasympathetic nerve, which dominates when a person is relaxed.

Additionally, the number of natural killer cells in their blood increased—these are the cells that attack virus-infected and certain cancer cells. City walkers showed no change in blood pressure or parasympathetic nerve activity.

Stress Reduction and Anxiety Management

Life, especially modern life, causes stress. Successful people across all walks of life seem to experience more than their fair share. The greater portion of any life success often seems impossible without hard work, pushing oneself and others, and meeting the demands of various situations. However, the responsibilities, frustrations, and pressures of daily life generate stress. This stress compromises wellness, particularly when accumulative, leading to physical resources running down while disease, injury, and accidents rise. Chronic stress can cause diseases, accidents, and other premature deaths, second only to smoking and alcohol as the leading cause of suffering and handicap in Western society.

Chronic stress interrupts thought and judgment, affecting mood and behavior. It interferes with mental clarity and emotional balance, erodes our sense of well-being, and exacerbates anxiety. It separates us from ourselves and our environment, making life unpleasant and often unbearable. However, the forest, in its full significance, offers beneficial effects on stress and mental strain. The harmony and beauty of fauna and flora, combined with the challenge and enjoyment of walking along a trail, serve as a distraction from the risks of inactivity and a sedentary lifestyle. Physical activity, aerobic exercise, movement, and calisthenic commitment not only improve cardiopulmonary function but also enhance musculoskeletal health, weight control, and vascular and coronary function. Hiking is one trailhead to ameliorating stress, with the forest opening wide to those who follow it.

Improved Mood and Emotional Well-being

Individuals suffering from depression, anxiety, and negative emotional states report decreased symptoms due to physical activity in natural settings. Green walking, such as along tree-lined paths, empty highways, and forest views, is particularly effective in treating anxiety and depression. This low-level physical exercise not only boosts physical health but also offers a cost-effective, risk-free alternative to medical treatments. Studies suggest that those suffering from mood disorders who are not yet ready to engage in physical activity can still benefit from passive contact with nature.

Accessibility to nature, especially a personal blue or green room, is crucial for mental happiness. For instance, having a water view from your property can be a significant asset for mental well-being. In such cases, the walkability of the community might do little to reduce stress. Instead, a secure, natural space can help minimize the likelihood of developing mental and physical disorders. Avoiding clear visual or physical access to pedestrians or cars can help residents feel safe and at ease.

The Social Benefits of Hiking

Hiking and being in nature bring specific social benefits, such as providing a common referent for conversation and turning small talk into meaningful dialogue. Whether with others or in solitude, the outdoor environment fosters open, significant discussions and promotes positive social relationships. Hiking creates feelings of goodwill and encourages positive social behavior. In contrast to the isolation often felt in small urban groups, small groups in nature experience their emotions collectively in response to the awe of natural events, such as spotting an animal, discovering a hidden spring, or encountering natural forces like a rainstorm or a bear.

Hiking can also promote altruism by fostering cooperation and unity within a group or community. The cooperation that emerges during hiking can benefit others globally. Hiking instills a sense of renewal, escape from the everyday, and adventure as we engage with living natural elements. These experiences are essential to each of us and bond us through shared experiences in nature. When people discover something stunning together and share its positive impact, it helps eliminate conflicts. Counselors can harness this common element to transfer positive experiences from individuals to groups, fostering meaningful connections.

Building Relationships and Social Connections

Social support is vital to good health. Being socially connected—having a network of close friends, family members, spouses, partners, or others to talk to, enjoy leisure activities with, and rely on in times of need—can significantly impact our wellness. Conversely, lacking strong social connections has been linked to poor outcomes, illnesses, and decreased life expectancy. Providing support for others can enhance our wellness by giving us a sense of purpose and helping us establish and maintain a positive identity. Balancing giving and receiving support and empathy is crucial.

Regular physical activity, such as walking or hiking, enhances our social connectedness and well-being by promoting relationships. The paths and trails of parks, forests, and gardens can serve as corridors to connect people, support family interactions, and encourage beneficial social support that contributes to health and longevity. Walking and being outdoors together can also strengthen relationships and enhance social connections. For example, couples often communicate more effectively while walking in a natural setting, as their bonding occurs in the presence of non-human factors. Walking together can reduce stress and depression, increase feel-good endorphins, promote positive interactions, and enhance happiness and relationship satisfaction.

CHAPTER 3

The Spiritual Benefits of Hiking

Going away to a quiet retreat or taking time to be alone in nature is a familiar ritual in many religious and spiritual practices. The ancients recognized the benefits of this practice for the spirit, as illustrated in the following parable found in both Christian and Buddhist tradition:

A young man came to live in a monastery seeking peace of mind and relief from the painful memories of war. He soon learned that the older monks spent long hours practicing solitude away from the monastic compound, often wandering for hours in personal study and contemplation. Curious, he asked the abbot why some brethren left each morning to hike alone. The abbot replied, "The journeys make them healthy." So, the abbot sent the young man off on the trail for a day. Upon his return, the abbot asked why he seemed so at peace. "You were wrong," the monk said. "Journeys do very little for health. But I believe I have discovered the answer to peace of mind."

The simple fact is that leaving the demands of our daily routines allows our long-range life perspectives to reset. Getting away from the constant irritants and pleasures that consume our immediate awareness helps put our successes and problems into more realistic proportions. This distance enables us to recognize that much of the conflict we often feel in our lives is not important. An awareness of the greater world, and our relatively small stature in it, can help put many of the usual problems into a clearer, less threatening light. The tranquility of nature sought by the monks is attainable through hiking. We all need this pathway to tranquility and heightened spiritual awareness.

Connection to Nature and the Sacred

The forest has long been revered as a sacred place, a realm of spirits and legends. Scientific research in Japan using fMRI scans of people looking at forest scenes compared to city scenes found that the brain was more relaxed around forests. Trials before and after spending time in the forest found that their parasympathetic nervous system—the part of the brain that controls relaxation—was enhanced while in the stillness of the trees. Touching the textured surface of wood can induce tranquility and ward off stress. Traditional cultures consider touching wood to be therapeutic—even seeing wood is relaxing. Researchers into forest bathing found that after years of searching for natural ingredients that combat disease and relax people, the most unusual of them all comes from the forest, specifically the forest air.

Psychologists Rachel and Stephen Kaplan propose that exposure to nature (what they call "attention-restoration") positively impacts humans. The quietness of natural environments transfers feelings of peace and comfort to individuals. Stress levels are reduced, allowing for uninterrupted meditation. Concentration becomes stable, emotional acceptance is enhanced, and spirituality deepens. Natural parks or forests tend to heal the body and spirit through their restorative forces. According to environmental and architectural theorist Peter Wohlleben, "even brief breaks in rural or forested areas" are "key to sustaining a healthy mind." Essential components of a natural place that promote tranquility include beautiful scenery, sounds from the natural world, and a multi-sensory environment with the movements of small and wild animals and flowing water. These experiences sensitize the senses and emotions, leading to the cessation of stressful thoughts.

Jacob let the silence settle once more, giving everyone time to absorb his words, to find the courage, if they wanted, to open up. He looked around the circle, his expression calm and encouraging. "If anyone would like to share something—about your loved one, about how you're doing lately, or anything at all—we're here to listen."

Elena felt her chest tighten as his words hung in the air, her eyes drifting to the floor. She could feel the quiet tension around her, the weight of unspoken words resting on each person. She wanted to speak, to say something about David, about the loss that had hollowed her out. But the words stayed trapped inside her, blocked by the fear of exposing her pain, of letting others see the depth of her vulnerability.

Across the circle, an older man cleared his throat, his hands trembling slightly as he adjusted the cap on his head. He gave a small, awkward smile before looking around, his gaze finally settling on Jacob.

"I lost my wife last year," he said, his voice barely more than a murmur. "After fifty-two years together." He paused, his eyes watering, and looked down at his hands. "There isn't a day that goes by where I don't reach over to her side of the bed, expecting her to be there." He chuckled softly, though there was no joy in it. "It's like my brain won't let her go, like some part of me still thinks she's coming back."

A ripple of understanding seemed to pass through the group, a shared recognition of that familiar feeling—holding on to someone who was no longer there, their presence lingering in small, everyday moments. Elena felt her heart clench; she had often done the same, finding herself reaching for David's hand in the dark, expecting his warmth to be there beside her.

Next to him, a young woman with a nervous smile raised her hand slightly, her fingers clutching the edge of her chair. "I lost my dad six months ago," she said, her voice soft, almost timid. "I still hear his voice sometimes, giving me advice. Telling me to be strong. I used to think it was weird, but now I kind of... I don't know... I like it. It makes me feel like he's still here, like he's guiding me."

Jacob nodded, his expression understanding. "That's a beautiful way to carry him with you," he said gently. "Grief isn't just about what we lose; sometimes, it's also about what we find—a way to keep our loved ones close, even when they're gone."

Elena felt a surge of warmth at his words, a reminder of David's gentle presence that she had felt in her dream, the echoes of his love lingering even after he had left her. She thought about the signs she had felt in recent days—the whiff of his cologne, the soft strains of his favorite song—and wondered if that was her way of carrying him forward, her way of feeling his love, even in the empty spaces.

Others spoke too, some sharing only a sentence, others delving into longer stories, each one marked by a rawness, a quiet vulnerability that made Elena feel both connected and exposed. Each person's story touched her, echoing parts of her own grief, each one a reminder that she was not the only one navigating this impossible landscape of loss.

As she listened, a part of her wanted to speak, to tell the group about David, about the beautiful life they'd built together, about the plans they'd made that now felt like fragments of a dream. But another part of her—a part she barely understood—held her back, clinging to her grief as though it were something precious, something she wasn't ready to let anyone else see.

She shifted in her seat, the urge to open up clashing with the instinct to remain silent, to keep her pain locked inside where it felt safe, untouched by the eyes of others. She wondered if sharing it would make it real in a way she wasn't prepared for, if speaking the words out loud would force her to confront the enormity of her loss.

Yet, as she looked around, she felt a quiet pull, a soft invitation that seemed to come from everyone in the room. Their stories, their willingness to sit with their own pain, made her feel a small flicker of strength. She wasn't alone; each of them carried their own sorrow, their own loss, yet they were here, bearing witness to each other's grief, a testament to the resilience of the human heart.

Jacob's gaze drifted toward her, a subtle encouragement in his eyes. He didn't say anything, didn't push, but the kindness in his expression made her feel that it would be okay if she chose to speak—or if she chose not to.

She took a shaky breath, opening her mouth as if to say something, but the words caught in her throat. All she could manage was a slight nod, a silent acknowledgment of his support, her way of saying thank you, but not yet. Jacob seemed to understand, giving her a reassuring nod before shifting his focus back to the rest of the group.

The session continued, each person sharing pieces of their lives, small fragments of the people they had loved, the parts of themselves that had been changed by loss. Elena listened, letting their words wash over her, feeling the weight of their grief mingling with her own. And though she hadn't spoken, she felt the beginnings of a connection, a sense of solidarity that softened the edges of her sorrow.

When the group fell quiet, Jacob glanced around, his eyes warm, patient. "Thank you, everyone," he said softly, his voice filled with genuine gratitude. "It takes courage to share, and it takes courage to listen. By being here, we remind each other that we're not alone in this, that we can carry our loved ones with us, even when they're no longer by our side."

Elena's throat tightened, the truth of his words resonating deep within her. She realized that, maybe, being here was her first step toward healing, a way to carry David with her without letting his absence consume her entirely. She didn't know if she was ready to speak yet, but being part of this circle, listening to others, was enough for now.

As the session drew to a close, she felt a quiet sense of gratitude settle over her, a small, fragile hope that whispered of new beginnings, of the possibility of moving forward without losing him. She hadn't spoken today, but maybe, in time, she would. For now, she was content to sit with her grief, to let it be seen, if only in the company of those who understood.

As she rose to leave, she felt the weight of her grief shift ever so slightly, as though the group had helped her carry it, even if just for a little while.

CHAPTER 4

Practical Tips for Safe and Enjoyable Hiking

Whether you're new to hiking or have been part of the hiking community for a long time, you might still have questions, issues, or concerns for your next adventure or for many future hikes. Here are some practical tips to help you along the way, whether you're standing still in a contemplative yoga pose or moving swiftly (but carefully) along a trail.

1. Know Your Ability and Fitness Level: Select trails that match your fitness level. Adhering to the "Three Golden Rules of Hiking" ensures your hike will be enjoyable. Remember to take regular breaks for rest and hydration.

2. Choose a Suitable Trail for the Group: When hiking with family or friends, it should never be about competition. Hiking should be an enjoyable bonding experience. Take the time to picnic, swim, or explore, considering the needs of the group. The smallest, the weakest, or the slowest will benefit the most and will cherish the experience. Embrace the slower pace, as it makes the memories even richer.

3. Prepare Adequately: Before heading out, make sure you're well-prepared. Pack essential items such as a map, compass, first-aid kit, snacks, and sufficient water. Dress in layers to adapt to changing weather conditions and wear sturdy, comfortable footwear.

4. Be Aware of Your Surroundings: Stay on marked trails to protect the environment and avoid getting lost. Be mindful of wildlife and respect their habitats. Always leave no trace by packing out what you bring in and not disturbing the natural surroundings.

5. Safety First: Inform someone about your hiking plans and expected return time. Carry a fully charged phone and, if possible, a portable charger. Know the signs of common hiking ailments like heat exhaustion or hypothermia and how to respond to them.

6. Enjoy the Journey: Hiking isn't just about reaching the destination; it's about enjoying the journey. Take the time to appreciate the beauty around you, from the small details like a wildflower to the grandeur of a sweeping landscape. Reflect, meditate, or simply breathe in the fresh air.

Hiking is an opportunity to connect with nature, improve your physical health, and strengthen social bonds. Follow these tips to ensure your hiking adventures are safe, enjoyable, and memorable.

CHAPTER 5

Choosing the Right Trail for Your Fitness Level

When you pick up any organized hiking guide, start by reading the introductory pages to gain valuable insight into the trail descriptions. Many guides use a rating system for trails, often breaking them down into easy, moderate, and difficult categories. For beginning or casual hikers, it's wise to stick to trails marked "easy." Many easy trails are located within or near campgrounds, making them accessible and perfect for a gentle introduction to hiking.

Your decision should be based on your current physical condition, not your intended future fitness state. It's important to know your ability and select trails accordingly.

Easy Trails: Easy trails are generally flat, gentle, and well-marked. These trails provide an excellent way to gently strengthen your entire body and stimulate your immune system, serving as a precursor to tackling more challenging trails. For instance, while the Appalachian Trail is known for significant elevation changes, even sections of it marked "easy" can help you lose weight and build stamina without overwhelming you.

Moderate Trails: Moderate trails offer a variety of terrain features and canopy experiences. They often include steeper inclines and more uneven terrain than easy trails. Forests at higher altitudes typically make for more challenging hikes than those at lower elevations, such as in Bradenton, Florida. These trails usually lead from developed areas into more remote wilderness, providing a balance between accessibility and adventure.

Difficult Trails: Difficult trails are best suited for experienced hikers in good physical condition. These trails often feature steep climbs, rough terrain, and longer distances. They require a higher level of endurance and preparedness. It's crucial to be honest about your fitness level and choose trails that match your abilities to ensure a safe and enjoyable hiking experience.

Practical Tips:

1. **Research and Plan Ahead:** Before heading out, research the trail. Understand its length, elevation gain, and difficulty level. Check weather conditions and prepare accordingly.
2. **Prepare Your Gear:** Ensure you have the right gear, including sturdy hiking boots, a map, compass, first-aid kit, sufficient water, and snacks. Dress in layers to adapt to changing weather conditions.
3. **Pace Yourself:** Start with shorter, easier trails and gradually work up to more challenging ones. Listen to your body and take breaks as needed.
4. **Stay Hydrated and Nourished:** Carry plenty of water and nutritious snacks. Hydration is key, especially on longer trails.
5. **Hike with Others:** Whenever possible, hike with a buddy or a group. It's safer and can be more enjoyable.

Hiking is a rewarding activity that offers numerous physical and mental benefits. By choosing the right trail for your fitness level and preparing adequately, you can ensure a safe and enjoyable hiking experience.

CHAPTER 6

Essential Gear and Equipment for Hiking

When getting ready to hit the trails, having the essential gear is crucial. Wearing the right clothing and bringing the necessary equipment—like food, water, maps, and safety gear—can make your hike more comfortable, legal, and safe. While hiking isn't difficult and doesn't require a lot of specialized gear, it's best to at least wear the right clothing and shoes, carry plenty of food and water, a map, compass, first-aid kit, and have a safe way to start a fire. While not necessary, a light daypack, camp chair, lightweight tarp, and trekking poles can add convenience and comfort to your hike.

Even on a casual short excursion, a hiker needs to bring water, food, a flashlight, and some type of navigation to avoid getting lost, and should wear the right clothes and shoes. Here's a breakdown of what to consider:

1. Clothing and Footwear:

- **Layered Clothing:** Dress in layers to adjust to changing weather conditions. Include moisture-wicking base layers, insulating layers, and a waterproof outer layer.

- **Sturdy Footwear:** Invest in good hiking boots or shoes that provide support and are suitable for the terrain.
- **Hat and Sunglasses:** Protect yourself from the sun with a wide-brimmed hat and sunglasses.

2. Navigation Tools:

- **Map and Compass:** Always carry a detailed map of the area and a compass. GPS devices and smartphones are helpful but should not be relied upon solely.
- **Guidebook or Trail Info:** Reading up on the trail beforehand can provide valuable insights.

3. Food and Water:

- **Hydration:** Bring sufficient water and a way to filter or purify additional water sources.
- **Snacks and Meals:** Pack high-energy snacks like nuts, dried fruit, and energy bars. For longer hikes, bring meals that are easy to prepare and nutritious.

4. Safety Gear:

- **First-Aid Kit:** A well-stocked first-aid kit is essential for treating minor injuries.
- **Fire Starter:** Carry waterproof matches or a lighter and a fire starter.
- **Multi-tool or Knife:** Handy for repairs and various tasks.

5. Comfort and Extras:

- **Daypack:** A comfortable backpack to carry all your essentials.
- **Trekking Poles:** Provide stability and reduce strain on your legs.
- **Lightweight Tarp or Shelter:** Useful for unexpected weather changes.
- **Camp Chair:** For added comfort during breaks.
- **Flashlight or Headlamp:** Essential for visibility if hiking extends into the evening.

Preparation Tips:

- **Know the Climate and Terrain:** Understand the local climate and terrain to dress appropriately and prepare for any challenges.
- **Plan Your Route:** Know the distance, conditions, and estimated time for your hike. Inform someone of your plans.
- **Check Local Safety Guidelines:** Be aware of any specific trail safety needs, seasonal considerations, and local weather patterns.

Proper conditioning and knowledge can make hiking in different seasons and locations enjoyable and safe. The goal is to be well-prepared without over-preparing either financially or physically.

CHAPTER 7

Nutrition and Hydration for Hikers

Hikers need a balanced diet that includes protein, carbohydrates, fats, vitamins, and minerals to fuel their bodies and maintain optimal health on the trail. Here's a breakdown of what to consider:

Protein: Protein supplies the essential amino acids needed to repair tissue damage, make red blood cells, and build hair and fingernails. While meat has traditionally been considered the best source of protein, plant-based sources like beans and nuts are now recognized as healthier options with fewer health risks. Healthy protein sources for hikers include low-fat dried meats, nuts and seeds, beans, and lentils. Although these plant-based sources might lack some essential fatty acids, they also reduce the absorption of fat-soluble vitamins A, D, E, and K. Hikers' higher ratio of fat to muscle means less protein is needed to prevent muscle-wasting, so it's possible to overdo protein.

Carbohydrates: Energy for hiking comes mainly from complex carbohydrates found in corn, oats, pasta, and whole grain breads. Blood sugar levels change more slowly with fiber-rich whole grains and vegetables packed with vitamins and minerals. However, many hikers have mismanaged their carbohydrate intake by carrying no bulky, slow-digestion foods and choosing white breads and sugary power drinks, leading to wild fluctuations in blood sugar and energy levels. Simple sugars like sucrose, glucose, and fructose work, but a sports drink or other concentrated carbohydrate forms are easier to carry. To maintain steady energy levels, opt for complex carbs and fiber-rich foods.

Fats: Fats are essential for long-distance hiking as they provide sustained energy. Unprocessed sources like seeds and nuts are best because the essential fatty acids are associated with proteins rather than sugar. Eating high-fat foods means less processing for a longer release of energy. However, it's important to balance fat intake with other nutrients to avoid potential health issues.

Vitamins and Minerals: A lack of essential nutrients can contribute to disease and poor health. It's crucial to consume a diet rich in vitamins and minerals to support overall health. Fresh vegetables and fruits are excellent sources of vitamins and minerals. For overweight and obese hikers, it's important to balance energy intake with nutrient-dense foods to avoid deficiencies and manage weight effectively.

Hydration: Staying hydrated is crucial for hikers. Carry sufficient water and consider bringing a portable water filter or purification tablets to ensure access to clean water. Sports drinks can also be useful for replenishing electrolytes, especially during long hikes.

Practical Tips:

1. **Plan Your Meals:** Prepare balanced meals that include a mix of protein, carbohydrates, and fats. Pack lightweight, nutritious snacks like nuts, dried fruits, and energy bars.
2. **Stay Hydrated:** Drink water regularly and monitor your hydration levels. Avoid waiting until you're thirsty to drink.

3. **Balance Your Diet:** Ensure you're getting the right amount of nutrients per calorie. Fresh vegetables and fruits should be a part of your diet to avoid nutrient deficiencies and skin conditions like lesions or scaling.

4. **Be Mindful of Medications:** Overweight and obese hikers may require more sugar and fat. Those with multiple medications should be aware of potential drug-disease interactions and allergies. Consult with a healthcare provider to manage medications and nutritional needs effectively.

Maintaining a healthy diet with the right nutrients per calorie can protect hikers from overweight, obesity, and skin rashes, saving hundreds of dollars per year and reducing medication management costs.

CHAPTER 8

First Aid and Safety Precautions

1. **Basic Knowledge:** Having a basic knowledge of first aid and safety precautions is essential for any hiker venturing into the woods. Emergencies are likely to occur at some point in a hiker's lifetime, and recognizing simple preventative safety measures can ensure a pleasant outdoor experience for everyone. This chapter provides the essential first aid and injury prevention knowledge that forest hikers need.

2. Hiker's Code of Conduct: Hikers have a code of conduct similar to the Hippocratic Oath of physicians or the ethical obligations of lawyers. This unique hiker's code of "do no harm" is crucial, and every hiker should uphold it. In the more remote, less-populated state and national parks throughout America, hikers are often the first responders to emergencies until park rangers and other volunteers can arrive. In such situations, minutes can mean the difference between life and death. Regardless of the location, the well-being of others and the protection of the environment should be the highest priorities.

3. Responding to First Aid Incidents: When a first aid incident occurs, stay calm and gather information about the patient's condition and the location of the incident. If you are the leader of the hiking group, assign specific tasks to those with you. This includes sending a runner to the nearest phone, instructing someone to administer aid and comfort to the victim, and asking someone to run back to a trailhead for help. Only those with medical training should evacuate any victim of the emergency. Keep others away from the scene unless they are providing direct assistance.

4. Safety Measures and Protocols:

- **Buddy System:** Always use a trail buddy system to ensure all group members return to the starting point.
- **Parking Lot Ticket System:** Use a parking lot ticket system to keep track of group members.
- **Preventative Measures:** Recognize and implement simple preventative safety measures to avoid emergencies. This includes carrying essential safety gear such as a first-aid kit, fire starter, and navigation tools.

By adhering to these first aid and safety rules, hikers can ensure a safer and more enjoyable outdoor experience. Whether you're a beginner or an experienced hiker, these precautions are vital for everyone in the hiking community.

CHAPTER 9

Environmental Awareness and Leave No Trace Principles

Leaving no more trace than your footprints is the first step in environmental awareness. Expanding our actions to prevent environmental damage is at the core of our sense of environmental stewardship. As an environmentally literate public, our collective task is to meet the environmental challenge head-on.

Unfortunately, too many hikers leave more than just their footprints behind. Though the impact from hiking is dispersed among many individuals over vast landscapes, making any one person's impact difficult to see, the cumulative effect is significant. If we don't take responsibility for our frequent intrusions into wild country, we can't expect the land to remain at its unspoiled best. Trails and natural environments are often impacted by "incognizant" hikers, diminishing the wilderness experience for everyone.

Leave No Trace Principles:

1. **Plan Ahead and Prepare:**
   - Know the regulations and special concerns for the area you'll visit.
   - Prepare for extreme weather, hazards, and emergencies.
   - Schedule your trip to avoid high-use times.
   - Repackage food to minimize waste.
2. **Travel and Camp on Durable Surfaces:**

- Stay on established trails and camp in designated areas.
- Walk single file in the middle of the trail, even when it's muddy.
- Avoid creating new campsites or trails.

3. **Dispose of Waste Properly:**
   - Pack it in, pack it out. Carry out all trash, leftover food, and litter.
   - Deposit solid human waste in cat holes dug 6-8 inches deep at least 200 feet from water, camp, and trails.
   - Pack out toilet paper and hygiene products.

4. **Leave What You Find:**
   - Preserve the past: examine, but do not touch, cultural or historic structures and artifacts.
   - Leave rocks, plants, and other natural objects as you find them.
   - Avoid introducing or transporting non-native species.

5. **Minimize Campfire Impact:**
   - Use a lightweight stove for cooking and enjoy a candle lantern for light.
   - Where fires are permitted, use established fire rings, fire pans, or mound fires.
   - Keep fires small. Use only sticks from the ground that can be broken by hand.
   - Burn all wood and coals to ash, put out campfires completely, then scatter cool ashes.

6. **Respect Wildlife:**
   - Observe wildlife from a distance. Do not follow or approach them.
   - Never feed animals. Feeding wildlife damages their health, alters natural behaviors, and exposes them to predators and other dangers.

- Protect wildlife and your food by storing rations and trash securely.

7. **Be Considerate of Other Visitors:**
    - Respect other visitors and protect the quality of their experience.
    - Be courteous. Yield to other users on the trail.
    - Take breaks and camp away from trails and other visitors.
    - Let nature's sounds prevail. Avoid loud voices and noises.

Conclusion:

The Leave No Trace principles provide a framework for minimizing our impact on the environment while enjoying the great outdoors. By following these guidelines, we can ensure that natural spaces remain pristine for future generations to enjoy. It's about creating a culture of respect and responsibility, ensuring that our wilderness experiences are sustainable and enjoyable for everyone.

CHAPTER 10

Hiking Etiquette and Respect for Nature

Everyone shares the trails, and everyone should exhibit common respect and consideration for others enjoying nature.

1. Choose the Right Trail: Some trails are heavily used to the point of being overused, while others are less frequented. When in doubt, opt for the lesser-used trail to reduce your impact on the environment.

2. Tread Lightly: Resist the temptation to pick flowers or feed animals. The goal is to leave the trail as you found it so others can enjoy it just as you have.

3. Stay on the Trail: Going off-trail can harm the environment and requires trail-finding skills. If everyone went off-trail, the forest would be needlessly trampled. Safety is also a concern—going off-trail can lead to injuries like twisted ankles or getting lost.

4. Extinguish Cigarettes and Build Safe Campfires: Always extinguish cigarettes properly and build safe campfires. Uncontrolled fires can cause significant damage to natural habitats.

5. Keep Dogs Leashed and Under Control: Dogs can disrupt wildlife and other hikers' experiences. They should be leashed and kept under control at all times. Remember, dogs do not belong in wilderness areas without proper supervision.

6. Don't Feed Wild Animals: Feeding wild animals is detrimental to their health and can be dangerous to humans. Wild animals are best left in their natural state without human intervention.

7. Never Drop Litter: Carry out all litter, including biodegradable items like food scraps. Leaving litter behind mars the natural beauty of the environment and can harm wildlife. The principle is simple: pack it in, pack it out.

Additional Tips for Respecting Nature:

- **Respect Wildlife Habitats:** Observe animals from a distance and do not disturb their natural behaviors. Be especially mindful during breeding seasons.
- **Minimize Noise Pollution:** Enjoy the sounds of nature and keep noise levels low. Loud noises can disturb wildlife and other hikers.
- **Respect Cultural and Historical Sites:** If you come across historical or cultural sites, appreciate them without altering or taking artifacts.

Conclusion:

By following these etiquette guidelines and respecting nature, we can ensure that hiking remains a pleasant and sustainable activity for everyone. It's about creating a culture of respect and responsibility, allowing natural spaces to thrive for future generations to enjoy.

CHAPTER 11

Hiking for Specific Health Conditions

Your stamina level required for daily hikes is determined by your physical health condition. Any unusual physical ailments or conditions should be referred to a physician for recommendations before beginning a hiking program. However, once you have received a physician's approval, the following information about hiking areas can greatly benefit your well-being and happiness.

When the ancient Greeks and Romans pondered how to live to a ripe old age, their recommendations included exercises such as walking in the hills. During the Golden Age of Health, approximately a century ago, the "placebo" effects were often reported through various natural remedies. One notable example is the Middle-Forks Ditch Trail, now known as the Stevens Trail in Whitewater Canyon, northeast of Auburn, California.

When I had pneumonia, my physician recommended hiking to benefit my lungs by increasing respiration and dilation patterns to enlarge lung capacity. Long hikes improved my condition faster than drugs and medication. Hiking exposed me to a form of natural air conditioning, and although I would often end a summer hike bathed in perspiration, I learned to change out of my hiking clothes promptly to avoid the risk of pneumonia. These combined conditions showed me that my pulmonary problems were minimized by daily physical exertion.

1. Hiking for Arthritis and Joint Pain

One increasingly popular, effective, and medically recognized method of controlling arthritis is light exercise. According to the latest health research, occupational therapists and other health professionals have found that walking is highly beneficial in managing arthritis and joint pain. For individuals with severe arthritis who are also obese, the simple act of walking can improve mobility and reduce pain, even when additional diseases like heart disease or diabetes coexist.

Regular activity is the fastest and most effective way to shed pounds safely. The good news is that you don't need to walk a lot to experience positive benefits. Any thoughtful, moderate movement program can contribute to effective arthritis reduction. For those overweight and afflicted with osteoarthritis, even modest amounts of level walking can be beneficial. For instance, Uttarakhand's trekking trails offer a natural, pine forest environment where a half-mile walk each day can burn as many calories as jogging twenty miles on hard surfaces.

An adventure in the Dehradun forest region can also include harvesting over sixty species of commercial, plant-based products used in Ayurvedic medicines, providing both physical activity and a connection to nature.

2. Hiking for Mental Health Disorders

Hiking is also recommended as an effective non-pharmacological therapeutic strategy for treating mental health problems. Patients with major depressive disorder, characterized by low self-esteem and depression, benefit from exposure to nature. Unconstructed open spaces create a sense of freedom, allowing movement through nature and helping increase self-esteem. Contact with nature gives patients vitality, reducing the intensity of their symptoms.

Nature walks can also lead patients to cognitively review their relationships with the outside world and increase their social support network. Studies have shown that the presence of water in natural settings enhances the therapeutic effect, reducing psychological symptoms.

The therapeutic effect of the forest on depression has been tested experimentally. Participants recruited through newspaper advertisements reported improved well-being after forest walks compared to town walks (control groups). Even if people cannot go outside, looking at actual nature, trees, woods, and green spaces offers restorative effects. There is a positive relationship between attentional abilities and the visual signs of restorativeness.

Hiking also offers a physically challenging activity that can reduce hostility and aggression. An experiment comparing the effects of walking in a natural arboretum versus a city arboretum found that walkers in nature reported less anger. This effect suggests that the stress reduction associated with simply taking a walk in a natural setting can significantly impact mental health.

CHAPTER 12

Hiking as a Therapeutic Practice

Hiking is clearly an exercise, but walking in nature is also a meditative practice. In meditation, we clear our thoughts, quiet our bodies, and feel the peace that comes from tranquility. In walking meditation, we are present in the moment, aware of every movement, and totally focused on what we are doing. Hiking offers all these possibilities and more.

It is well known that more and more hospitals are offering "forest bathing" to cancer patients as a therapy to promote health and happiness. The high content of the aroma substance α-pinene, a long-lasting balsamic odor found in forest air, can enhance the immune system's fight against disease. In Japan, many people deliberately breathe in forest air in special parks called "shinrin yoku," and Japanese scientists have proven that the immune system strengthens during time spent there.

An Australian research study from 2003 documented the healing power of green spaces, calm woods, sweet-smelling flowers, trickling water, twittering birds, and gentle wildlife. Participants in this survey reported an increase in their immune defense. Kansas University professor B. McGary of Recreation, Park, and Tourism Sciences found in his own 2014 survey that perception and medical value comfort the mind and heart, enhance mental and emotional states, foster personal growth, and improve cognitive functions. The risk of serious diseases was lowered, and injuries and pain were less considerable. Worship songs as social support also filled the mind, giving rise to physical and psychological self-care. This theory has been verified by many medical scientists multiple times.

Ecotherapy and Nature-Based Interventions

Ecotherapy, also known as eco-psychology or nature therapy, is a rapidly growing field in therapeutic applications and community-based interventions. It acknowledges the importance of the living environment on the health of individuals and communities, based on the person-environment interaction model. It combines attention to both the inner and outer landscapes. Nature-based interventions are often affordable, accessible, and engage people actively in a non-medical or non-pharmacological environment. Nature stimulates our sense of wonder and curiosity. The idea is to partner with our non-human family members to absorb some of the benefits of a nearby forest adventure, whether a simple nature walk or a multi-day hike.

Nature-experience quality matters, and specific guidelines on how to optimize nature-related interventions might be necessary. Non-clinical individuals might benefit from preventive nature interventions in public health, whether through community greening programs or direct experiences in nature-based educational projects. It's not just the physical activities (such as walking) that impact an individual's sense of wellness but also the social interactions and sense of community. This may be part of the power of a community that shapes attachment and a sense of place within a neighborhood, leading to a more natural and sustainable way of life.

Forest Bathing and Shinrin-Yoku

Forest bathing and shinrin-yoku are deeply embedded in mind-body wellness, harking back to ancient health practices of the Greeks and traditional Chinese medicine. Stepping outside into nature is both preventative and curative to one's health. Today, walking in the forest is identified as a leisurely way to maintain vitality, uplift the spirit, tone parasympathetic nervous function, and revitalize mental energy.

The essence of forest bathing lies in the forest atmosphere, such as airborne substances, the surface of the earth, the soil, and the rich fragrances from trees and flowers. The healing powers found in fresh air, water, sunshine, and birdsong play a significant role in affecting humans in therapeutic ways. Participants in forest expeditions often show positive and statistically significant changes in their emotions of happiness and relaxation. Reducing and decreasing stress and anxiety through these experiences brings calm, happiness, and energy. Creating a connection between the human heart and the heartland is a therapeutic practice that promotes overall well-being.

CHAPTER 13

Case Studies and Success Stories

Case study: Outsmarting MS on the Appalachian Trail

Debra's story is truly inspirational. Debra had been an active person who loved the outdoors. A diagnosis of MS had slowly taken over her body and left her feeling defeated. She wanted more than anything to prove everyone wrong and show that she still had the strength and resilience that was such a huge part of her. At the end of 2012, Debra decided to go against the odds and through-hike the Appalachian Trail. Once she made the decision, she committed herself to a journey of wellness. She trained her body the best she knew how. She put together a support team. She went on the walk of a lifetime. The author had the pleasure of being one of Debra's trail angels. The lasting effect she left on all of those who reached out to support her was amazing.

Debra's "Outsmarting MS on the Appalachian Trail" has taken the wellness journey and turned it into a phenomenon. Knowing Debra and her determination, I fully believe that she has changed many people's mindsets for the better. It is easy to make excuses for all of our (not so good) habits or laziness, but it is awesome to see someone prove them all wrong in such a huge way. Debra's journey has only made me realize that with a little more energy and effort, I can do so much more. I am fulfilling the life she knew and loved. I am inspiring myself and sharing the story of a wonderful woman who fought back with vigor and gained so much in the process. Citizens nationwide followed her via the documentary "Trail Magic: The Grandma Gatewood Story." This was created to honor the legacy of an ordinary woman who peacefully hiked an extraordinary amount of miles on the Appalachian Trail, stunning the country and world in the process.

Personal Transformation through Hiking

No matter what our state of health might be at any given period in our lives, the experience of engaging in a healthy physical activity is profoundly and emphatically satisfying to our mind and spirit. When we take specific steps to improve our state of health, to beat back an addiction or compulsion that may be slowly destroying our mental, emotional, and physical health, we become stronger and forever changed and strengthened at our core. Daily difficulties and struggles are met easily and with more confidence, a purpose-driven life unfolds for us unclouded by the entangling demands of diseases. A decision to hike for health's sake can be the first step in a community or effort to reform both our mental and spiritual selves.

Depending upon the nature of our determination, our hike might simply be a peaceful morning stroll or clutter our lunchtime with various geological, historical, and natural discoveries. We might, too, change careers, open a health resort, cultivate an herb farm, and promote the benefits of natural wellness centers. People come to such places, often at the end of their strength, for healing of mind, body, and spirit, a peaceful time for exactly that essence. It becomes an essential ingredient for ripping the busy, stressful bomb's mouth out of injured lives at their roots, and for that always removed back to the placid, healing aspects of days. Each personal re-solve strengthens the resolve of others, allowing them also to find and make their way.

Conclusion: Embracing the Healing Journey on Fores

Increasing numbers of individuals should consider hiking as part of a holistic approach to health, incorporating both preventative healthcare and healing therapy. Hiking offers numerous benefits with few side effects, no prescription necessary, and individualized dosages. Healthcare providers, including doctors and nurses, should advocate for spending time hiking on forest trails. However, this recommendation should be personalized, accounting for each individual's medical history.

As hikers return to the forest, the concept of treatment can be reframed as "forest medicine," highlighting the beneficial effects of aesthetically pleasing landscapes and their impact on a person's inner well-being. The widespread acceptance of the psychological benefits of scenic natural areas, such as forests, will likely lead to increased efforts to protect and manage these environments, making them conducive to recovery and healing.

Recognizing nature as therapeutic on forest lands emphasizes the medical and ethical considerations that support this notion. Embracing hiking as a holistic health practice can help individuals connect with nature, improve their physical and mental health, and promote a deeper appreciation for the natural world. This, in turn, fosters a greater commitment to environmental stewardship, ensuring that future generations can also benefit from the healing power of nature.

By integrating hiking into our health routines, we can embark on a healing journey that nurtures our bodies, minds, and spirits. Let nature be your guide, and allow the forest trails to lead you toward a healthier, more balanced life.